RELIEVE YOURSELF OF PAIN AND IMMOBILITY IN JUST 7 WEEKS OR LESS

Here's How The Lives Of Two NHS Nurses Suffering From Excruciating Pain And Immobility Was Changed After ___ ___ How You Can F___

Debbie Shi
RN Dip HE, Dip MT (MC)

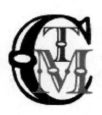

MTC Publishing

First published by MTC Publishing in Derbyshire, UK

ISBN 978-0-9556588-0-8

Catalogue Data
Shimadry, Debbie
Relieve yourself of pain and immobility in just 7 weeks or less: Here's How The Lives Of Two NHS Nurses Suffering From Excruciating Pain And Immobility Was Changed After Just Weeks and how you can find relief too/ Debbie Shimadry.

1. Health 2. Alternative Therapies 3. Self help

MTC Publishers provide books on alternative health, for more information or to speak to a qualified alternative practitioner write to or call:
MTC Publishing,
Unit 6, Karlsruhe House,
18 Queens Bridge Road,
Nottingham,
NG2 1NB
U.K
Tel: 0800 612 1346

CONTENTS

Introduction

Let's face it: when a nurse or doctor contracts arthritis or back pain—or any other chronic complaint—they turn to modern medicine for help. Sometimes they find that conventional medicine can't help, even after years of attempting to. As far as conventional medicine is concerned it's the end of the story for those people, apart from taking even more painkillers.

This happened to two NHS nurses, who even with their exhaustive knowledge of traditional medicine, were unable to find anything that could make one bit of difference to their pain and suffering. They were left, after years of medical attention and treatment, with virtually no mobility and pain at such a height that it certainly indicated to them that conventional medicine had no answers for their problems.

This is where two experienced NHS nurses Debbie Shimadry RN Dip HE Dip MT (MC) and Dee Parsons RN Dip MT (MC) decided to make one final effort to resolve their excruciating pain and immobility. Frankly, neither of them believed one little bit that what they did was going to work... but it was a last ditch effort.

To their utter surprise and delight, they found that their pain quickly began to dissolve—and their mobility also quite quickly began to be restored. In fact, within just 7 weeks both nurses had virtually completely lost their pain and also regained practically complete mobility.

This flew in the face of all their training, and everything they had learnt in the whole of their combined NHS experience. But it worked, and that's all they cared about—and that's probably all _you_ care about too.

The likelihood you are reading this book is because you have a degree of pain and immobility. Maybe it's slight, may be it's severe—or maybe it's crippling. **My answer to you is that I can't offer you better advice than to give clinical magnetic therapy a try.**

Let's move on now to the story. I think in these pages you will find a solution and a way out of the pain and immobility your are suffering. There's no need to suffer it a day longer in our experience.

Read on. I think you will enjoy—and more important—the likelihood is that you can benefit for the rest of your life.

Chapter One

When Conventional Medicine Failed To Find A Solution For Two Of Its Long Time NHS Nurses, They Had To Take A Leap Of Faith As A Last Resort-Effort To Resolve Their Pain And Immobility

Here's how myself and another NHS nurse—who couldn't be helped by conventional therapy—discovered and used clinical magnetic therapy to relieve our pain and regain our mobility. The other nurse happens to be my mother.

My mother Dee suffers from osteoarthritis which has infiltrated into her back, knees, hips, feet, hands, shoulders and neck. In January of 1999 she became so debilitated by her condition that she became unable to walk.

In brief, the bones in her feet were simply crumbling away. Every step was excruciatingly painful. Dee couldn't walk or drive or even leave the house. Her arthritic pain started 19 years ago, and it started in her neck with headaches. The doctor said it was stress, and suggested relaxation. The headaches continued, and then the pain spread down into the neck and all the way across her shoulders.

She went back to the doctor twice a week every week to ask for help with the pain. Dee suffered with the pain in her neck and her shoulders— plus had a permanent headache for months. She was at the end of her tether, when she went to see a friend, and told her all the symptoms she was feeling. The friend recommended going to see a chiropractor, who was finally able to determine what was wrong. He could tell that it was Spondylosis. She started on massage treatment—which did help to a degree—but she needed twice-daily massage to keep the pain at bay.

Dee's back pain started when she was 14 years old; she endured terrible pain through her entire spine right the way through her teenage years. The doctor always put it down to 'growing pains'. At the age of 21; Dee was convinced that she couldn't still be experiencing 'growing pains'. Finally, investigations revealed that she had Spondolythesis in her spine—and the specialists could offer no treatment except permanently wearing a wide, hard and very ridged back brace.

Ultimately in 1999, her many different joint problems completely took control of her life, and she had no choice but to give up nursing, on sick leave. As she became 100% housebound, unable to go upstairs, drive, or even walk her dog 100 yards—in fact she couldn't leave the house. All she was given to take were anti-inflammatory and painkillers. Neither had any helpful effect whatsoever.

My own story is slightly different. I fractured my spine in two places 16 years ago in a horse-riding accident. I was enjoying a relaxed, leisurely trek with a few friends in September 1991, when disaster struck for me.

. My horse was startled by a bird. Suddenly he lurched to the side, and as he did so, he tripped on a rock. I, unable to hang on, flew over his head and crashed to the ground with a tremendous thud... and snapped my spine in two places.

A&E X-rayed my back, and couldn't see the fractures. It wasn't until eight weeks after that they realised their mistake. I was still suffering intense pain and wasn't able to bend down or twist. I seemed to be permanently at the G.P's office and got the impression that he was utterly sick of the sight of me.

I felt that I had no choice but to ignore the constant the pain, trying desperately to get my life back to normal, but there were so many things that I still couldn't do; the pain restricted all my movements. Plus I would wake up as many as 15 times every night in agony, and would have to manoeuvre myself to the edge of the bed and then inch by inch slide to the floor and—on hands and knees—try to release the rock-hard muscle spasm which caused by back to stiffen.

Getting out of bed in the morning was a whole different kettle of fish. Honestly it looked like a scene from a comedy sketch, and I guess it would have seemed funny to me if it wasn't for the gut-wrenching agony that accompanied it. I eased myself across the bed at a snail's pace; then came the debacle of rolling over onto my stomach, hanging my legs over the edge of the bed, kneeling on the floor and eventually working myself to the end of the bed... where I clung onto the bedstead for dear life as I hauled myself into and upright position. After this 15-minute fiasco I would have to slowly stretch my spine gently until I could feel my vertebrae unfreezing.

My work as a nurse didn't help because I was constantly lifting and moving patients. I also had three young children, (which as you can probably imagine!) only served to degenerate my spine condition further.

Over the next year I tried acupuncture, massage, exercise, physiotherapy and osteopathy to no avail. During this time, an osteopath revealed that my spine had twisted itself into an S shape and—as a result—my pelvis had become unhitched on the right hand side. He got me to side on the couch and stretch my legs out in front of me, and I started in utter amazement as one of my legs was three inches longer than the other. He explained that because my pelvis was unhitched, I was completely lopsided... and that was why my legs looked different lengths.

It was Dec 1999 when I hit absolute rock bottom. Just two days before Christmas, I was lifting my eldest child (then 4) out of the bath... when my back just 'popped'. By 10pm I lay on the bed unable to move at all. The next morning, Christmas Eve, I called my osteopath. As soon as he saw me, he confirmed that I had slipped a disc. He advised me to lie on my side, put ice packs on, and come back after Christmas.

I spent Christmas day lying on the sofa with a bag of frozen peas stuck down my knickers. I ate my Christmas dinner alone on the sofa whilst everyone else enjoyed the festivities at the table. Words can't describe how thoroughly miserable I was. That year my New Year's resolution was to find an answer to my never-ending suffering.

In early 1999 I, like my mother, found myself essentially housebound and on crutches... unable to work, drive or even pick up my children.

Then, a chance and last-resort discovery provided a very unexpected solution...

The last-resort discovery was clinical magnetic therapy. The promise from the person who suggested it was reduced swelling, increased blood flow and reduced pain... and best of all it was completely natural.

Frankly, had Dee and I not reached this last-resort situation, we never would have believed it enough to try it. But, and particularly because it proved to be completely natural and safe, we thought, "lets give it a go for at least a few weeks."

Truthfully, as professional nurses we had great doubt that something this simple could have any meaningful effect. But we had nothing to lose.

Here's what happened next: we were both as astonished as each other. After 5-7 weeks we were relieved of all pain, and regained our mobility.

Dee found that the pain in all affected areas—knees, hips, back, hands, neck, feet and shoulders—had completely (not just partially) gone. She was able to walk again; she was able to bend and reach up again. In short, her life was restored.

The same happened with me. The pain, which I suffered for 16 years because of my riding accident simply seemed to dissolve away over 6-7 weeks. And I regained virtually all my mobility and ability. I was once again able to pick up my children, do the housework, drive the car and go to the gym. The magnets haven't cured my back—I still have the abnormality there... But what they have done is take away all the pain and swelling.

I went back to my nursing position in Intensive Care and life was virtually—maybe not 100% but 99%—returned to normal. I look forward to each day now instead of getting up with a sense of dread. I've lost so much time being miserable and in pain. Now all I want to do is live life to the full with my family—who had to put their lives on hold as well. Now there's no stopping us!

As you can imagine—and especially because we are both nurses—with a desire to help people, heal people and see people through the misery of pain and disability, we couldn't wait to share this proof with as many people as we could.

Within months, we formed an organisation whose purpose is simply to make available this extraordinary clinical magnetic therapy to as many people as we can reach. And that is the majority of people who are suffering from pain and immobility due to the following debilitating ailments:

- Osteoarthritis
- Rheumatoid Arthritis
- Osteoporosis
- Fibromyalgia
- Spondylosis
- Polymyalgia Rheumatica
- Spinal Stenosis
- Disc Prolapse
- Multiple Sclerosis
- Stroke
- Peripheral Vascular Disease

Relieve Yourself Of Pain And Immobility In Just 7 Weeks Or Less

- Diabetic Neuropathy
- Leg Ulcers

That's what we've been doing since 2001. Here are some of the results that we have achieved since then:

Out of 10,773 people that we have treated, 10,018 have reduced their pain and substantially increased their mobility. Plus 6,511 have been able to reduce the amount of pain killers they take each day, and 2278 no longer require any painkilling medication.

There is so much unnecessary pain and unnecessary lack of mobility. Our main purpose is to get as many people as possible to experience reduced pain and increased mobility.

Obviously medicine is the first and most important port-of-call, and as nurses we understand that and we agree with it.

However clinical magnetic therapy is very interesting, and something that is possible for people in pain and suffering with a lack of mobility. When medicine has given up, there is something else that can help.

Perhaps when medicine has reached the limit of what it can do for your pain—you would be willing to open the door—and at least consider whether clinical magnetic therapy can help you in the same way it helped and continues to help us.

Chapter Two

How It Works: The Science Behind Clinical Magnetic Therapy

Chinese, American, Russian, German and UK scientific studies have discovered that sufficiently strong magnets (not fridge or toy magnets) placed over and around an injury reduces pain and swelling.

The magnetic field created by placing magnets around your area of pain, which is completely safe and harmless, penetrates through your skin and into the muscles and tissue surrounding your injury, causing pressure on your nerves to be released and your pain to subside.

What's more, the same magnetic field stimulates the production of more red blood cells around your area of pain. This provides a rich, fresh supply of oxygen and healing nutrients to your area of pain.

Most importantly, the blood carries a vast amount of endorphins (hormone); your body's natural painkillers; directly to where your pain is.

Absolutely <u>NO</u> Side Effects

You will not feel any ill effects from clinical magnetic therapy. It does not alter the way your body works.

Very simply, it stabilises and realigns your body, allowing it to heal the injured area it is placed around.

And remember, clinical magnetic therapy is 100% non toxic, drug and chemical free, and entirely harmless.

Plus, you are perfectly safe to use magnets if you take prescribed or non prescribed (supplements) medication.

They do not interfere with any tablets, regardless of how many you consume each day or what they are. You will be completely safe using clinical magnetic therapy.

The Facts Are These:

About 63% of users of clinical magnetic therapy are able to significantly reduce the amount of painkillers they take. 35% no longer need any painkillers at all.

The correct clinical magnetic therapy treatment is a breakthrough in pain-management and relief, with the added important benefit of physically freeing immobile joints.

Quickly, I Want To Reassure You About Just One Thing:

If you are suffering with pain and immobility right now, you genuinely can reduce your pain by at least 50 to 75%, and in many cases by 100%.

- Even if you have had your pain for countless years,
- Even if you are severely physically restricted by your pain,
- Even if you have a multitude of other medical conditions,
- Even if you take a handful of tablets each day,
- Even if you have tried just about everything, and nothing has worked for you.
- No matter what age you are—the oldest person we have treated is 97.

And most importantly, it works on all types of joint, muscle and circulatory related conditions. In fact, all of these conditions can be helped:

How It Works: The Science Behind Clinical Magnetic Therapy

- Osteoarthritis
- Rheumatoid Arthritis
- Osteoporosis
- Fibromyalgia
- Spondylosis
- Polymyalgia Rheumatica
- Spinal Stenosis
- Disc Prolapse
- Multiple Sclerosis
- Stroke
- Diabetes
- Peripheral Vascular Disease
- Diabetic Neuropathy
- Leg Ulcers
- High blood pressure
- Migraine
- Insomnia
- Repetitive Strain Injuries
- Tendonitis
- Carpal Tunnel Syndrome
- Bowel Disorders

Let Me Be Crystal Clear:

You cannot compare magnetic therapy with anything you have tried before. It does not work in the same way as any of these treatments:

- Tens
- Acupuncture
- Reflexology
- Osteopathy
- Chiropractic

Relieve Yourself Of Pain And Immobility In Just 7 Weeks Or Less

- Massage
- Physiotherapy
- Steroid Injections
- Nerve Blocks

If you have tried any of these treatments and they haven't resolved your pain, magnetic therapy can still work for you.

The Relief Of Your Pain Starts Immediately

Clinical magnetic therapy begins its work the moment you first place it on, and as you keep it in place day and night.

It will only be a matter of 3 to 6 weeks on average before you begin to feel either a significant or total relief of your pain.

What will happen is this: as the magnetic field starts to reduce your inflammation (swelling) and increase your endorphin levels, you will begin to regain mobility in your joints, and movement will be easier. Over a period of days or a few weeks you will feel the benefits gradually increase.

The saddest thing I hear and see is people suffering from pain and mobility restrictions, and not knowing about magnetic therapy.

My greatest wish is that you will find your pain-relief through this incredibly simple, gentle and yet vitally effective clinical magnetic therapy treatment.

Incredibly, people who have been severely physically restricted are able to be almost 100% active again; gardening, enjoying family activities, travelling, playing sports, walking their dogs, and shopping within just a few weeks—even as short as a week or two—after using clinical magnetic therapy.

Chapter 3

I Call It A Miracle—The Power Of Clinical Magnetic Therapy

Historically it is reported that magnets have been around for an extremely long time. Magnets were first documented around 2500–3000 BC. Their origins are first noted in Asia Minor in a vast land called Magnesia. The earth there was enriched with iron oxide, which attracted metals to it. The locals named it Magnetite.

Another story is told of a young boy, who lived in 2500 BC, called Magnes, a shepherd on Mount Ida. One day he was tending his sheep whilst wearing sandals, which contained iron rivets in the sole. He found it hard to walk up the mountain, as his feet felt heavy and stuck to the rock face.

Mount Ida was found to contain a rock called lodestone, which is the first known magnetic mineral. It is reported that lodestone was named Magnes after the boy who discovered it, and it later came to be known as magnet.

Cleopatra was probably the first celebrity to use magnets. It is documented that she slept on a lodestone to keep her skin youthful. The therapeutic knowledge was passed to the Greeks who have been using magnets for healing since 2500 BC. Aristotle and Plato talked of the benefits of lodestones in their work.

Magnets have been used in Chinese medicine from around 2000 BC in conjunction with reflexology and acupuncture. It is still used today as a first-line treatment for many common complaints.

Relieve Yourself Of Pain And Immobility In Just 7 Weeks Or Less

3,500 years after they were first discovered, magnets have gained popularity in Europe and the USA. In the 15th Century a Swiss physician named Paracelsus recognised the therapeutic powers of magnets. He wrote medical papers on the influence of magnets on the inflammatory processes within the body.

In the 16th Century an English doctor, Dr William Gilbert, made a scientific study of electricity and magnetism. He published one of the first books about magnetic therapy called "De Magnet". Dr Gilbert was also Queens Elizabeth I's personal physician, and it is said that she used magnets under his direction.

Michael Faraday, also known as the founder of Biomagnetics, made extensive discoveries in magnetic healing during the 18th Century. His work is still used as a framework for modern-day magnetic treatments. Dr Franz Mesmer (the father of hypnotism) and Dr Samuel Hahnemann (the father of homoeopathy) also contributed to his remarkable work.

20th Century pioneers include Dr Kreft, a German doctor who in 1905 studied the healing effects of magnets on rheumatic disease, sciatica and neuralgia. 1926 revealed Dr Criles' work on the impact of magnets on cancer cells, and this was followed 10 years later in 1936 with Albert Davis carrying out tests on the effects of the North and South poles of a magnet.

However the last 15 years has shown a prolific increase in medical research into magnetic therapy. There have been over 57 studies in the USA into incurable diseases and magnetics. Some of the most recent are:

1990—University of Hawaii tested magnetic fields on patients with osteoarthritis.

1992—Stiller, et.al. conducted a randomised double-blind trial of wound healing in venous leg wounds.

1999—New York Medical College tested magnetic insoles on diabetic patients.

2001—University of Virginia tested magnetic mattress covers on patients with Fibromyalgia.

2004—University of Exeter and Plymouth tested magnetic bracelets on patients with osteoarthritis.

Magnetic therapy is gaining in popularity worldwide, with many celebrity devotees including:

- Cherie Blair
- Bill Clinton
- Anthony Hopkins
- HRH Prince Charles
- HRH Prince William
- HRH Queen Elizabeth II
- Shirley Maclaine
- Venus Williams
- Michael Jordan
- Andre Agassi
- Jack Niklaus and many more.

Here's How Clinical Magnetic Therapy Conquers Pain

You simply wear clinical magnetic therapy devices directly over the area of pain.

They are soft and stretchy, comfortable to wear, and contain extremely lightweight and small clinical-grade magnets (not fridge or toy magnets).

The clinical magnetic therapy straps or jewellery are designed to fit almost anywhere on your body.

NOTE: regardless of where your pain is, and what type of pain it is, there is <u>one rule</u> that applies to all types of pain: <u>Clinical Magnets must be placed directly over the area of pain to have an effect.</u>

Relieve Yourself Of Pain And Immobility In Just 7 Weeks Or Less

Unfortunately you cannot treat the whole of the body with just one magnet. And that is because of a very simple principle of physics (you may have been taught this at school):

Think of your skin as a pond or lake, and then imagine the magnetic field as a stone being thrown into the lake or pond. At the place where the stone entered the pond, the ripples are very strong, tightly-bunched and close together. As the ripples move out across the water, the ripples get further and further apart and become weaker.

Exactly the same happens with the magnetic field when you place it on your skin. As you move away from a magnet, the magnetic force decreases. What this means is when you place a magnet on any point of the body, the magnetic field is at its strongest right at the point of contact with the magnet and the body. The further the magnet is from an area, the weaker the magnetic field.

For example, if you placed a 3,000 gauss magnet on the wrist, the magnetic force around the wrist would be 3,000 gauss, but 4 cm away from the wrist the strength is only 187.5 gauss and at 8 cm only 46.88 gauss.

This principle is known as the Inverse Square Law. You don't have to memorise this law to be able to use magnets effectively, but it is very important to understand that the further away a magnet is to the point of injury, the weaker the magnetic field will be. This is why magnets should always be worn directly over (or as close to as possible) the point of injury.

In short: wherever the pain is located, you must place magnets within that area or within very close proximity.

Wear your clinical magnetic therapy straps or jewellery <u>day and night</u>. Only take them off to wash, and then put them straight back on again.

Clinical magnets must be worn 24 hours a day and 7 days a week to gain the maximum pain-relieving benefits. Every time you remove them, you are taking away the very device that is reducing your swelling, improving your blood flow, encouraging new cell growth, killing pain and freeing up joints.

The straps or jewellery should be worn next to the skin, but if you are sensitive to synthetic fibres such as elastane or nylon you can wear them over a very thin layer of clothing such as a vest or slip.

Your body heals by the greatest degrees at night whilst you sleep; it makes perfect sense when you think about it. When you're asleep your body shuts down all of its non-essential functions so that it has a surplus supply of energy. That excess energy is then used to accelerate the healing process. Hence, most of your body's healing work is done when you are sleeping. Plus, whilst you are sleeping, your body's immune system is replenishing itself and gaining strength.

Because you are asleep your organs do not need so much oxygen. This allows the body to concentrate on repairing the damage caused by inflammation inherent to chronic disorders.

When you sleep on a clinical magnetic sleep-pad throughout the night, the magnetism is very rapidly absorbed into the tissues and bloodstream, thus aiding the body's natural nocturnal healing process which is much quicker than during the day.

This dramatically boosts your body's natural healing process, reducing the time it takes for your pain to be resolved. In all honestly, night-time is the best time to use clinical magnetic therapy.

How To Drink Water That Is Amongst The Purest On Earth Just Like The Romans Did In Their Spas

The reason Roman spa water was so beneficial was because it was drawn straight from the earth (by tapping natural underground springs).

The natural magnetic field of the earth was imbued into the water. The natural spa water carried the magnetic charge, and it was absorbed by the water. That's what made it so beneficial health-wise.

Here Are The 8 Health Benefits Of Drinking Water That Has Been Imbued With The Same Natural Properties Of Roman Spar Water

1. Detoxifies and eliminates excess fluid which is stored in the body
2. Creates an abundance of energy
3. Induces deep and restful sleep
4. Safely and naturally reduces blood pressure (including high blood pressure)
5. Regulates hormone levels including serotonin (manages depression and mood), melatonin (a lack causes insomnia), endorphin (the body's own painkillers) and insulin (regulate blood sugar levels)
6. Calms and soothes bowel irritation and inflammation
7. Aids digestion and absorption of nutrients from food
8. Reduces inflammation in tissues and joints

You can emulate the purity and benefits of Roman spa water with a clever little device called a Water Wand.

Here's How The Water Wand Works:

It duplicates the magnetic field that the earth produces naturally. You simply place the wand in tap water and it magnetises (ionises) the tap water with the same magnetisation that spring water has, simply returning your tap water back to the way Mother Nature intended you to drink it.

Just 4 glasses a day is enough to see quite dramatic differences in your pain levels, but it can't be used alone; it must be used in conjunction with magnets directly over the area of pain.

I Call It A Miracle—The Power Of Clinical Magnetic Therapy

It can't harm you, and does not interfere with any medications or treatments. It does not alter your body in any way—it's simply natural water made as spring water again.

When you drink water that has been magnetised, the magnetism travels into the stomach and is absorbed into the bloodsteam through the bowel wall. It is then very rapidly distributed around the whole body.

Of course, the magnetic field that is circulating around the body has the same effect on the inside as the magnetic field has on the outside of the body. It will reduce inflammation within the body, plus increase blood flow and oxygenation of the tissues, especially around any damaged areas.

Think about it: when you drink magnetised water you are tackling your problem from inside and outside at the same time. This 2-sided approach will most definitely increase the strength of the magnetic field at the point of pain; plus it will also speed up the healing process by increasing the absorption rate of the magnetic field by an amazing 6 to 10 times.

Why The Water That Comes Out Of Your Tap Does Not Have Any Of The 8 Health Benefits That Pure Roman Spa Water Has:

In order to fully understand how magnetised water (Roman Spa water) works, it is important to know a little bit about the water that comes out of your tap.

The original source of water is mountain streams, which flow into rivers and eventually out to sea. As the water passes underground (many rivers and streams pass underground), it comes into contact with the earth's magnetic field. The magnetic charge is absorbed by the water, and it becomes magnetised. Similarly, as the water flows overground, it comes into contact with magnetic rock (lodestone) and water is again magnetised.

Once water is collected for consumption, it has to be treated and purified. During transportation to the treatment plant the water is carried in underground metal pipes. The water is de-magnetised by the presence of the metallic lining of the pipes, and when it is purified and comes out of the tap, it is no longer magnetised.

If you drink water from a spring at its source, it will be magnetised. The benefits of spring water have long been recognised, however once the water is bottled and removed from the source, it will only keep its magnetism for up to a maximum of 3 days before it dissipates. It is not possible to permanently magnetise water.

Why Roman Spa Water Is Different And More Beneficial For You Than Tap Water

Water seems, at first sight, to have a very simple molecular structure, consisting of just two hydrogen atoms attached to an oxygen atom. Indeed, there are very few molecules that are smaller or lighter. Once a water molecule has been exposed to a magnetic field, (the same magnetic field that is present naturally in the centre of the earth) the molecule changes in several ways:

The water molecule increases in size, by a fraction, but this increase makes a huge change in the water's solubility and permeability (the ability to disperse and penetrate other substances). What this means is: magnetised water improves your body's absorption of water as well as several other water soluble nutritional substances.

When the size of the water molecule is increased, its ability to absorb toxins is enhanced. Your body stores harmful toxins with in the tissues (dermis) of the skin. To keep the toxins from poisoning the body, they are stored in small pockets of fluid. This is seen as cellulite, and feels like lots of little raised bumps (the body can store an extra 2 litres or 4½ pints of fluid containing toxins in the tissues).

As magnetised water increases the size of the water molecule, its ability to absorb toxins is much greater. So, when the magnetised water is absorbed into the bloodstream and transported around the body, harmful toxins are drawn out of the tissues and safely carried to the liver, and then onto the kidneys for excretion from the body.

In a nutshell, you can lose as much as 2 litres (4½ pints) of excess unwanted fluid that you don't need. The knock-on effect of losing this excess waste fluid is that you will have so much more energy, plus you will feel less tired. Sleeping will become easier and generally, you will have a great sense of wellbeing.

Magnetised Water Sounds Like A Panacea For All Illnesses And Ailments; It Certainly Kept The Romans Healthy, But It Does Need To Be Used In-Conjunction With Clinical Magnets Placed Over The Area Of Pain

Magnetised water has numerous benefits for the body, and it will boost the strength of externally-used magnets by 6 to 10 times.

But when used alone, it will not take all the symptoms of an ailment away without any other magnetic devices. This is to ensure that the magnetic field that is circulating around the body has the same effect on the inside as the magnetic field has on the outside of the body

We discovered that this double-approach increases the strength of the magnetic field at the point of pain, and significantly helps to reduce pain quickly.

If you drink the odd glass of wine, just put your wand into your glass or bottle and you will taste the difference. Interestingly, with red wine, many people say that you can watch the wine becoming clearer over the period of an hour. Try it and see!

People who live in hard-water areas most often comment that their water tastes much softer and better. There is a softening action from the magnetic field in exactly the same manner as placing a large magnet on the outside of your water supply to reduce limescale deposits in your kettle, hot water tank and washing machine.

You CANNOT overdose on magnetised water because the magnetism is simply clearing and softening the water. This is why magnetism is used to stop limescale on your water pipes and it works. It has the same kind of effect in the body; it clears away toxins and refreshes and stimulates the blood flow. You can drink as much as you like.

The one thing you cannot do with your magnetised water is boil it, as the heating process destroys the magnetism. **Your magnetised drinks must be cold!**

Chapter Four

The 5 Additional Health Benefits You Gain Almost From Day One Of Using Clinical Magnetic Therapy

Clinical magnetic therapy also:

- Improves your circulation
- Encourages deep, long and restful sleep
- Maintains a toxin-free body
- Induces an abundance of energy
- Strengthens your immune system

How? In layman's terms, clinical magnetic therapy speeds up blood flow and causes several things to happen in your body:

Firstly, your circulation is improved. Basically the blood flows around your body more effectively, so you get more oxygen and nutrients to your organs, muscles, joints and limbs.

Secondly, clinical magnetic therapy will help to balance your hormone levels. What this means is the hormones insulin, serotonin, endorphin, and melatonin will be more readily-available and better regulated. When your melatonin (the hormone which induces sleep) levels have regained their optimum concentration, you will enjoy a deep and restful sleep.

Thirdly, the magnetic field aids the body in realigning the positive and negative ions which are present in every single cell. Your cells are like little batteries, each with a positive and negative end. If you put batteries in your radio the wrong way round, it simply won't work. The same principle applies to your cells.

Magnets push the cells back into perfect alignment so that any excess fluid and toxins are forced out of the tissues and flushed out of the body when you go to the toilet. You can "wee" up to 2 litres of unwanted, excess, toxin laden-fluid once you start using clinical magnetic therapy

Fourth, the combination of your increased circulation and the elimination of toxins will allow your heart to take a rest. You will have less fluid to push around your body and your blood will be flowing much more efficiently. This means your heart will not have to work so hard. Your blood pressure and pulse rate will <u>naturally</u> begin to lower, and you will feel a tremendous boost in your energy levels. In a nutshell, you will have a terrific feeling of wellbeing.

Lastly, the cumulative result of more oxygen, more nutrients, balanced hormones, and a rested heart is a strengthened immune system. You will be less likely to catch "bugs" and viruses. You will be able to fight infections better, and ward off coughs and colds. Your immune system protects your body from attack and harm. To protect your body, your immune system must be strong and healthy.

Chapter Five

Free Of Pain At Last! — 69 People Share Their Stories

I wanted to share these 69 stories with you because the facts are that 7.7 million people in UK suffer with arthritis and 16.8 million suffer with back pain—yet they don't have to suffer with the pain and immobility.

Let me share the experiences of these 69 people who all have had their pain relieved and their mobility restored with clinical magnetic therapy:

⁂

"I was in so much pain and I couldn't sleep in bed. I had to sleep sitting up in a chair. I bought the mattress cover and now I can sleep in bed. The pain in my shoulders and back has eased so much I can move about much better and I can sleep better and feel that I have much more energy."

"I couldn't sleep at all but now I can go to bed and sleep through the night. The water wand has really detoxified my body and increased my energy levels. My Fibromyalgia will never go but now it's manageable. My life was on hold and now I have it back."

"I used to ache all over, every fibre of my being hurt and it restricted me from doing the things I love the most, like gardening. I was even having trouble sleeping. But I can honestly say that using the magnetic mattress cover, wand and pillow has been marvellous. Even after just weeks of use I could feel the difference."

"When you have suffered for a long time and you suddenly have freedom from it, it's fantastic—and of course getting back out in the garden has been great. It has completely changed my life."

Liz Roberts

"I put the cover on my bed and started sleeping on it. I have been getting cramps in my legs and pain across my back, but I found that over this last week or so, I've lost the cramps. I don't wake up in the night with them now. My back is a lot better and I'm able to use my thigh muscles better to walk with. I can get in and out of the car easier and that's just in a couple of weeks. You must try these things; it's worth everything if it gets rid of the pain."

Bert, aged 84

"I was very sceptical to begin with. I didn't think that they would work for me. I bought a mattress cover a couple of months ago and believe me, it has really helped me in getting out of bed in the morning. The difference it has made is incredible. I'm not stiff anymore in the morning. I just get out of bed without any pain and it's wonderful. It really has helped me a lot and I can walk without a walking stick now; it's wonderful. I would be devastated if I didn't have my mattress cover, I couldn't face it and I'm sure I would be in a wheelchair now if it wasn't for the magnets."

Angie, aged 59

"The most striking effect that magnets have had in my life can be seen in the greatly improved movement of my feet. I have been wearing magnetic insoles for quite some time now and have watched my feet come alive again over the past months. It had become difficult to walk on anything but a really flat surface like a supermarket floor. Even slightly lumpy ground hurt my feet. Foot colour has improved due to better circulation.

I no longer notice the slight puffiness of my ankles; I move a lot better generally on my more flexible feet. Thank you for helping me so much."

N. French

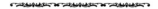

"For the last 8 years I have suffered from a very rare syndrome called 'Stiff Man Syndrome'. It is a neurological condition that effects muscle control, causing muscle spasms, rigidity and pain. The condition causes my speech to slur and I have difficulty in forming words. In April 2000 I lost my power of speech altogether. I had to communicate via a typewriting speech box. I was not very optimistic about my chances of success with magnets as there were no reported cases of treatment for Stiff Man Syndrome with magnets. However I was desperate and agreed to give it a go. I used the bar magnets and the pillow daily and the results were extremely impressive. The facial spasms have completely resolved, plus totally unexpectedly my speech returned.

I can't describe how life-changing the effects of the magnets have been to me. I was once again able to express myself. I have continued to sleep on the pillow pad, but I removed the bar magnets from my face. After regaining my speech for 13 days, I became unwell and my speech again deserted me. I immediately replaced the bar magnets and within just 2 hours the spasms had stopped and my speech returned. I have periods where I feel very well and my speech is perfect, but I also still suffer from relapse.

Overall I feel that there has been a tremendous improvement to my condition within the last 6 months. Since using magnetic therapy I have had perfect speech for 46 days within the last 6 months, compared with 9 days of speech in the previous 6 months without using magnets. Thank you all so very much."

Vanessa, aged 51

Relieve Yourself Of Pain And Immobility In Just 7 Weeks Or Less

"I am pleased to tell you that I have obtained much relief after using magnet therapy. The pain is almost gone from my right knee and I am walking a lot easier. I have always used the magnet around my knee in bed at night-time. I find this the easiest way and I shall continue using it this way."

M. Morgan

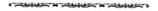

"Some time ago I was in constant pain from my right knee, with osteoarthritis. I could not do anything; shopping was limited and I needed an escort. But then I purchased a knee band and within a very short time I was able to move about freely on my own. Most of the pain disappeared and I could sleep at night. People told me how much I had improved; they said that it showed in my face. I have regained my confidence to do things I had given up doing; thanks to the band. It has saved me having an operation. So it has been money well spent from my point of view; well worth it."

L. Cook, Derbyshire

"We think the magnets are fantastic. My stiff and painful neck and shoulder is virtually better thanks to my necklace. My husband's distorted and arthritic finger is nearly straight thanks to his ring. The cat and I are enjoying a good night's sleep with the pillow insert."

L. Carnell, North Yorkshire

"About a year ago I broke my wrist, leaving me with a great deal of discomfort and swelling, which resulted in not being able to do household chores very easily. I was introduced to magnets and I purchased a strap for my wrist, which has greatly reduced swelling and freed me from pain. I would recommend it to anyone to help with pain relief."

E. Wass

28

"About 10 months ago, after a foot operation to realign the heel bones, I started having painful swelling on my hands, between the thumb and wrist. It was very painful; especially the right hand—when under any sort of pressure. My back was also uncomfortable in the lumbar region, so gardening and bed making etc became a trial. On having a check up, I was told that my blood pressure was up and my hands were arthritic. However, at this very same time I saw an article in our local paper from World of Magnets.

So all to gain and nothing to lose, I sent for the information pack and made an appointment for Dee to phone me. My queries were answered and encouraged. It made a difference knowing that you have experienced these ailments. The results so far are that, to start with, I was taking three ibuprofen tablets each day; last week at my check up, I have been taken off the ibuprofen. It still hurts sometimes but the inflammation is gone and my blood pressure is returning to normal; though I'm still on the tablets.

This is after wearing a Monet bracelet day and night for 3 weeks and drinking lots of magnetised water. My hands still hurt sometimes if I 'do too much', but seem to recover more quickly. I think that it is very likely that using the magnetic bracelet has saved me from becoming a chronic case. My husband has just sent for a pair of your magnetic insoles. This must be praise indeed for your magnets!"

Margaret W, aged 74

"I've had no problems with my neck since I started sleeping on the mattress cover and pillow. I haven't had one bad day since I started sleeping on it. I usually get struck down by a chronic fatigue that takes over me and I have to just go to bed for days on end. I can't remember the last time that I had to do that.

It has made a huge difference to my life. I live on 5 acres and have to tend animals and since using it I haven't had a single day where I have not been able to get outside and do things. I'm delighted it's made such a difference to my life."

Celia Dennison

❦ ❧ ❦ ❧ ❦

"I decided to use magnets to try and help my fibromyalgia, which caused me pain in many areas of my body, including my head neck and shoulders. I started to use a magnetic pillow and a water wand and within 7 days I started to feel a difference. I now sleep better at night and have more energy."

M. Dobson, aged 55

❦ ❧ ❦ ❧ ❦

"I met Dee at a ladies' group where she spoke about magnet therapy. Since a child (I am now 80) I have suffered with rheumatism so decided to give it a try. After choosing a bracelet, pillow and mattress cover, I found after 10 days that I could get my engagement ring on over my knuckle; the first time for several months. Also since using the pillow and mattress cover (which is very comfortable) I've been sleeping more soundly and haven't had to get up during the night to go to the toilet. My energy levels have also certainly improved, especially in the mornings. At my age you can not put the clock back but magnet therapy seems to be helping me."

G. Fellows

❦ ❧ ❦ ❧ ❦

"I do not know if 'thank you' is enough; after I felt so ill and depressed with a blood pressure of 195/85. After a consultation, you advised a water wand and bracelet, which I received the next day. Just three weeks of this magnetic wonder I feel fine; blood pressure down to 147/67. Wonderful."

H. Johnson

❦ ❧ ❦ ❧ ❦

"As a youngster I had a sporting life; racing was my big passion and due to spills on and off the racecourse I've broken my ribs, shattered my left arm at the elbow and right collar bone and of course the hips take a pounding when bouncing down the race track. Now with age I suffer with a lot of aches and pains and stiffness; which I did until I was introduced to World of Magnets' products. I wear a magnetic necklace for the relief of my stiff neck and enhanced mobility and a magnetic bracelet which has relieved my right elbow of the constant pain. I also use a knee magnet support. I can't thank World of Magnets enough for the relief their products have given me."

Rod

"I have had arthritis in my wrist and fingers for several years. Due to the swelling I have been unable to wear a ring of great sentimental value to me, having previously belonged to my dear mother.
I am so pleased now. After wearing the hematite bracelet for only 6 weeks, I am able to wear my ring again with great pleasure."

Kathleen

"Two years ago I had surgery to rectify sciatica. Unfortunately I got an infection in a disc which resulted in more than 2 months of immobility due to intense pain. My back was constantly aching, restricting my movements. One morning I heard about World of Magnets on the radio. I phoned and spoke to Dee. She recommended the new bed pad and water wand. After using them for a week, my back felt stronger and the aching was dramatically reduced. Five weeks of therapy, and I continue to feel improvements—and I'm beginning to enjoy my life again."

M. McNicholl.

"I have suffered with frozen shoulder for nearly 5 years. I could not lift my arm sideways without experiencing a lot of pain, which increased as my arm got horizontal. The pain got so bad that I couldn't lift it anymore. I read about magnets in our local paper, so I thought I'd give it a try with a shoulder support. Within 24 hours of wearing it, I could tell the difference.

Relieve Yourself Of Pain And Immobility In Just 7 Weeks Or Less

Within a month I could touch my ears with my arm with hardly any discomfort. I only wear it at night now. The shoulder strap for me is better than sliced bread—marvellous! I would recommend it to anyone."

Sam Becket, aged 57

"I am writing to say how grateful I am to World of Magnets. Some years ago I had a bad fall injuring my leg, ankle and foot. I had X-rays and tests for many months, then I was told they were unable to help me. The veins in my leg and ankle were damaged and my foot was twisted. I was given a support for my leg, but it only kept the swelling down. I was in a lot of pain, unable to go out or do my housework. I was told about magnets by a friend. I brought a knee band and ankle strap. Within two weeks, I was having less pain, sleeping better and able to go out and do my housework. And now I take very few pain killers. I shall always be grateful to you."

O. Mecmans

"Within seven days of receiving magnets from you, the pain had gone out of my arm and shoulder. I had this pain for 3 years. I also sent for knee magnets and they have helped with the pain in my knees by fifty percent but it has not completely gone. So I would like very much to recommend that anyone with a problem tries using magnets as they have made me feel a lot better. Also thank you very much for all your assistance and help. It is a comfort to know that I can call you anytime should I need to.

M. Hallam

"I have for many months now been wearing one of your stainless steel bracelets. I suffer from both RSI and Carpal Tunnel Syndrome on my dominant hand. On wearing the bracelet for a matter of days, my ability to type for extended periods was enhanced by 50 to 70%. I could not stand the pain after prolonged periods at the keyboard. The effects were measurable because I recently lost the bracelet and the pain returned; there was a pro-

32

found difference between wearing it and not."

M. Eames

"My mother had a painful left hand and blue fingers due to bad circulation. Now after wearing the magnets for two weeks, most of the pain has gone and her fingers are back to normal. The back-belt was for me. I have had back pain for over 20 years. I had constant back ache. After wearing the back belt for some three weeks now, my pain has been reduced and the constant ache has gone away. Also my sleeping has got a lot better."

D. Groom

"I bought a magnetic pillow a year ago to help with my migraines which I used to get quite frequently. Since using my pillow pad, I have only had two migraines in the last year. I am sure the magnet pillow pad has helped. Thank you."

Mrs Clarke

"I first heard your broadcast on BBC Radio Lincolnshire. I was very impressed with what you had to say and your obvious enthusiasm for magnets. I took down the details and contacted you. My husband purchased a bracelet and has worn it ever since! As you will know I have purchased a double shoulder wrap, back belt, pillow and 2 pairs of shoe insoles - all have made a difference to us!! We are both chronic arthritis sufferers but feel we have benefited from these items."

E. Naylor, Doncaster

"I had a badly broken leg some years ago and had many problems with arthritis, swollen ankles, and knee and leg pain. I was told to try the magnets and was advised to have a water wand, insoles and a pillow. I have used them regularly and have found a significant improvement all round and in my general health. The level of support has been excellent from all the staff."

C. Scott-Ison

"I couldn't get upstairs because of my arthritis. After 4 weeks on the mattress cover all my pain had gone. I stopped taking my pain killers and I no longer need my tens machine. I certainly have more 'get up and go' and have managed to get back in my garden again."

Jean, aged 75, (Osteoarthritis)

"I wasn't sure whether magnets could ease my all-over body pain. I took the plunge and bought a mattress cover. Astonishingly after 2 nights I was sleeping through out the night. It's brilliant. I no longer wake up at all, having to change my position…I can't live without this mattress cover."

Tina, aged 54 (Fibromyalgia)

"I was asked to participate in a trial in magnetic therapy. I was given a small pad to put in the bed. I lay with my hip, which was my worst area of pain, on the pad every night. It was only small but it did take all the pain away from my hip and I thought I would need a much bigger pad because I've got pain everywhere. I was really very impressed with the test pad so I decided to go for a mattress cover.

It was brilliant. It did just what it said it would and my husband—who didn't want to use it—found that it helped with the arthritic pain in his knees. I even took it to Hungary with me on holiday. It's not a cure for my Fibromyalgia but the wonderful thing is that it constantly refreshes you through the night and it has really helped me so much more than I can say. I'm thrilled to bits with it. It has saved my life. It's well worth the money that you spend on it."

Vivienne, aged 67

My Dad had a mattress cover from you. It had been on the bed for 2 days and the pain in his back has gone and he is walking a lot more!!!! Thanks."

S. Lawrence

"I would just like to say how happy I am with the mattress cover I purchased from you 9 months ago. Since then I have been free from much of the pain I was experiencing when I came to you. I have recently seen the specialist at the hospital and found not only to have Fibromyalgia but also osteoarthritis together with spondylosis in my neck. I was in so much pain when I came to you and very frustrated by the side effects the drugs were creating with my stomach, together with the lack of sleep I was experiencing. I really was as you would say, at the end of my tether.

Thankfully, with the mattress cover I feel the situation has been helped. I am now getting a relaxed and pain free sleep. I have several customers suffering similar complaints and have highly recommended this cover to them; which I feel has made a vast improvement to my life and even saved me from giving up my business. It is wonderful and has been washed over and over again and still is just like new. Thank you—at least 99% of the time I can honestly say that I manage without the medication, and am still much of the time pain-free or at least the pain is manageable!"

J. Hodgson, Derbyshire

"Thank you for introducing me to the world of magnet therapy. Until now I have endured years of pain and discomfort following multiple surgical procedures on wrists, arms and elbows. I have been resigned to constant severe pain but now after only 2 weeks of using a magnet I can honestly say that I feel much better; by at least 50% or more. I can now see a light at last and hope for the future. Thanks to the magnets, I am beginning to enjoy my life now. I was very sceptical of new methods of pain relief, but not anymore. It works, and it is better for me that I am in contact with professionals who are helping me understand how it works. Once again thank you for showing me a different world than I've had for years."

Christine, aged 56

"The mattress cover was the turning point for me. I am over the moon. I have got my life back again. I can walk now. I get up in the morning and I don't feel achy all over and I'm so sprightly. I sleep much better now."

Janet Hutchings

"My back is a lot better than it was. In the last fortnight I have been aware that I haven't had any pain. I am sleeping on the bed cover every night. I am so pleased with my progress in such a short time."

Gloria Simons

"Since sleeping on the mattress cover for just 3 weeks, my pain has reduced by 90%. It's just sore now, when compared with what it was before. I think it's brilliant; it's worked much better than I anticipated. I am sleeping better at night and I can now walk for over an hour without pain. My joints are no longer troublesome and the muscle pain has almost disappeared completely. Thank you all so much."

Frank Smith

"I was in so much pain from my Fibromyalgia that I couldn't sleep in bed. I couldn't lie down; my shoulders were so bad that I had to sleep sitting up in the chair. I bought the mattress cover and it has really eased it. I can sleep in the bed now.
I find that it's not just beneficial to me, but also to my husband who was having trouble. He has arthritis in his back and he used to wake up with

back pain every morning. He has said how much difference it has made to him. It really has done us both good."

Carol Elks

"I've been using my magnets for a month now and they really are starting to have an effect. About a fortnight ago I realised that I wasn't waking up at night with any aching. I didn't ache in the morning either. It's great; thanks so much."

Noreen Lem

"The magnets have definitely helped me because I made a point of leaving them off for a few days. It was such a relief to put them back on again. The pain had come back with a vengeance.

At first you think that magnets are one of those things that you try for a few weeks and then chuck away. But until you actually try it you don't realise what it can do for you. It really has made my life a lot better."

Cath Jones

"My back and knees are a lot better. There is quite an improvement in my sciatica. I don't get the burn down my leg and I'm sleeping better as it's not waking me up in the night. It was awful before but now it's improved so much."

Mrs Anderson

"After just 2 weeks of use there seemed to be a big jump in my improvement. The magnets seem to be working well. I've got so much more flexibility. Before, when I woke up, I couldn't bend to put my trousers on until I had been in a hot shower. I've got the flexibility to do it straight away now.

Relieve Yourself Of Pain And Immobility In Just 7 Weeks Or Less

My feet were so stiff they cracked and banged when I got out of bed. They've improved no end. I'm pretty sure that I'm on the road to recovery now."

Ron Hind

"I've had Fibromyalgia, lower-back pain and sciatica for 30 years. I've been to osteopaths, chiropractors, had acupuncture, homeopathy and taken various tablets. I was very fed up and depressed. In May I heard about clinical magnetic therapy. I was sceptical that a magnet could help me but, out of desperation, I decided to try it.

Six weeks later my back has improved immensely. My headaches and whiplash injury is so much better. I can't believe the improvement. I am not depressed now, I can walk better and I am gardening again. I can do a lot more now than I could before trying the magnets."

Brenda Astling, aged 75

"I have suffered for the past 20 years with arthritis and Spondylosis. A friend of mine showed me some information on clinical magnets. Usually I would have thought 'what a load of rubbish'. But I thought to myself this time I would have a go. The first thing I tried was a pillow. After 2 to 3 weeks I was sleeping 3 to 4 times longer than I had previously; thanks to the pillow. I then plumped for the back belt, which I can say once again between 40 to 50% of the pain seemed to go.

I also started drinking magnetised water. I thought this will be a waste of money; 'it won't work'. But once I tried it, after about a week, I noticed a vast difference, just by drinking this special water. I then used a necklace for my neck pain and a strap around my knee; both have showed a big improvement. I can honestly say it's all been a huge success. These magnets are just marvellous. I can't believe it's true. Every word of the information I was given about clinical magnets was true.

I then went the whole hog and got a mattress cover to see if it made an extra difference. YES, YES, YES is all I can say. It made the world of difference, giving me even more sleep. I'm almost back to the way I was in my youth all those years ago."

B Altoft, aged 67

"I was suffering with back and neck pain after a car accident 5 years ago. I had had physio after the accident which lasted for about 6 months and was taking painkillers and anti-inflamatories. I had also started seeing a chiropractor and having regular massage, which I have not had to have for a month now because of the magnets. I used single magnets for months without much success; there was some pain relief but they kept falling off.

I decided to try a magnetic back belt instead and felt the relief almost immediately. I am now sleeping much better as I don't wake through the night like I used to. The pain has not completely gone, but has reduced it enough for me to stop taking the pain killers. I am still trying to take things easy as strenuous activities tend to make my back stiffen up, but even that has improved.

The other day I was doing some gardening and my back became so painful I could not move. I continued to wear my belt overnight and the next morning the pain had gone—which would have normally taken at least a week to subside. I am amazed at how this really does work!"

L. Higgin, aged 52

"When my pain was really bad I took paracetamol. I had pain in my ears, my wrist, head, shoulders and my arms. I decided to try various magnetic devices to help me, I had a ring, a bracelet, a necklace, earrings and a water wand, which I tried for 8 weeks.

Within an hour I could feel the difference. My headache and my shoulders were already benefiting and my shoulder pain was completely gone within 3 to 4 days. My wrist pain improved and after 3 to 4 weeks the pain is almost gone. I still get pins and needles sometimes, but not as bad as before. I used to wake up during the night in pain with my carpal tunnel syndrome; this got to be very painful and was waking me nearly every night. Now I have very little pain and I hardly ever wake during the night. I still get slight pain in the mornings but that is all."

Nancy Carrigan, aged 48

"I suffer with spinal stenosis and sciatica, which causes me pain in the lumbar region of my back, my thighs and my calf. I had tried 12 weeks of acupuncture and was taking paracetamol and brufen daily for 6 weeks with little effect. I then started taking co-codamol and then diclofenac, but during this time my pain has got worse.

I started to use magnets shortly after this in October. I used a magnetic back belt. In November I also started using a bed pad and drinking magnetised water. Within three weeks of using the belt, there was a 50% reduction in my pain and in December I managed to walk for 1 mile without any pain whereas previously I could only manage 100 yards. I can now walk up to 5 or 6 miles without any pain. In fact the only pain I feel now is a slight back ache first thing in the morning."

C. Wignall, aged 79

"Due to a car accident I suffered with lower back pain. I have also developed osteoarthritis and osteoporosis, which also caused me pain in my neck and back. I was taking paracetamol and ibuprofen before I tried magnetic therapy. I had also tried Physiotherapy and Acupuncture. I try to keep fit and healthy as best I can, which I love to do Tai Chi and Pilates for.

I had heard on the radio about magnetic therapy and decided to telephone for some information. I had already used a magnetic bracelet for some years but was advised to try a water wand and a bed pad. I was amazed at how much I improved, I felt the difference with 7 days.

I now have a mattress cover and certainly feel much better. I no longer take ibuprofen and only occasionally take paracetamol. I am not completely free from pain, but I certainly feel able to straighten up my body. I do stretching exercises to get going in a morning, but then I seem to forget about aching limbs and get on with my life; it's great. I have told family and friends who do admit a difference in me."

C Wilkinson, aged 71

"My pain was in many of my joints, ankle, knee, neck, spine, both wrists, elbow and shoulders and I had to take a lot of painkillers to just cope. I started with a small magnet on my ankle but then got a knee strap, water wand, insoles and a mattress cover. Within days, the pain had reduced in all areas. Now I'm only using the magnets, except for the insoles which I still wear during the day. At night almost all my pain is gone. I can now exercise my ankles and knees and shoulder without pain. My balance has improved, making going up and down stairs so much safer. I'm sleeping much better and have given up paracetamol and ibuprofen completely. I certainly have more energy and plenty of 'get up and go', now that I am almost pain free."

J. Prout, aged 75

"My arthritis affected my hands, my left knee and my lower back. The fact that I also suffer with an under active thyroid gland was an added problem. The pain was quite bad, and as a I couldn't exercise much I had put on a lot of weight, which was making the arthritis worse. I was taking diclofenac and tramadol and also had physiotherapy. I had tried an alternative therapy before, Acupuncture; but that didn't give me any relief at all.

I decided to get a magnetic mattress cover and a pillow pad and within 5 days I had noticed the difference. There was definitely a reduction in my pain. 6 weeks after that, the pain had almost gone. In January 2006 I decided to get a back belt and a knee strap to wear during the day and I started drinking magnetised water.

I sleep well now, and most of the pain has gone completely. I'm decorating my home again and gardening. I can now enjoy walking my dogs twice a day but still get some slight pain in my lower back. I am sure this is due to my obesity, but I am losing weight now, owing to the exercise—which I could not do before wearing the magnets. To be pain free most of the time is wonderful; life is now worth living again!"

M. Beckwith, aged 65

"I suffer with pain in my neck and back caused by arthritis. I have also had high blood pressure for many years. I was taking painkillers and seeing a chiropractor. I decided to purchase a magnetic mattress cover. There was some gradual improvement over a period of 3 weeks, but I then went on holiday without my mattress cover. When I got back it was good to get back to my mattress cover.

I really feel that as I continue to use the cover I will carry on improving with time. I feel much more free now and having more time with it will, I know, help me. For the first time in many years my blood pressure was 'spot on' according to the doctor. I feel it is the use of magnets that has achieved this. I know my age means that I ought to expect pain but since my husband passed away, I take pride in keeping the house and a large garden in good shape. I am a very active person and with the help of magnets I intend to continue to be!"

A Warren, aged 74

"I have arthritis in my joints and it mainly affects my fingers and thumbs, my knees and my shoulder. I did take painkillers, but only when I needed to as I didn't like taking too many. My fingers were getting worse and had started to become stiff. I looked into trying magnetic therapy and used small individual magnets placed onto the area that was painful. After 7 days there was a slight reduction in my pain, but after 3 weeks I am now mainly free from pain. It does return slightly from time to time, but my knees are completely free from pain."

J. Sharrock, aged 76

"I have suffered with arthritis of the spine since 1974 and had to wear a spinal corset for many of those years. Because of being unable to move so easily I ended up putting on weight and had to finish work. I now also have pains in my neck and feet and suffer with high blood pressure. I take brufen, codeine and paracetamol for the pain and decided to try magnets to see if they could help me.

I tried a magnetic bracelet, back belt and insoles and have had them for 5 weeks now. I now have had some pain relief from my shoulder and my back. I have no trouble sleeping now and am even managing to do my own shopping. I have passed on this information to my friends and family who are now interested in magnets for themselves!"

D. McCluskey, aged 82

"I suffer from sciatica, Spondylosis and diverticulitis which causes me pain in my neck, lower back, buttocks and legs. I had tried osteopathy and was taking co-codamol but I was still suffering with my pain. I tried a magnetic back belt first—which was good—but I felt I needed more magnetism. So I changed my back belt for a magnetic mattress cover and a water wand.

Within 14 days I had noticed the benefits and now after 2 months the pain has almost disappeared. My diverticultis pain has almost gone as well. The benefits are enormous for me and my wife who suffers with many ailments which have quite severely disabled her, one of which is spinal stenosis. She used to have an electric blanket on the bed all the time, even during the summer sometimes, but she no longer uses it any more. I have also purchased a small magnetic knee strap for my Father, and his knee is considerably better. I bought my Mother a magnetic necklace for her Spondylosis which is also much improved. I thoroughly recommend everything that I have tried. Thank you; they're very good products and well worth every penny!"

M. Gadd, aged 52

"I suffer with Carpal Tunnel Syndrome and lower back pain; I also get pain in my shoulders and in my fingers. I was having physiotherapy and taking paracetamol but it didn't really help. So I decided to give magnetic therapy a try. I purchased a water wand, a back belt and a bracelet at first and within 28 days there was a big reduction in my pain. Within 4 months all of my pain had gone. I decided to get a magnetic mattress cover to treat the whole of my body. My back pain has gone, except for a slight twinge occasionally. I sleep a lot better at night and I have resumed walking again. I have now gone back to doing my own gardening and decorating!"

M. Clegg, aged 67

"I bought two magnetic bracelets 3000 gauss, one last August and another about a month later, and by Christmas the pain in my hands, particularly the thumb joint and the first finger joint had dramatically improved. I then only needed to take the occasional Ibuprofen 400mgs tablet.

I went on a Caribbean Cruise for two weeks in March/April this year (2007), and had to keep renewing my cruise card as I couldn't get into our cabin. Eventually after the forth new card I realised that the magnetic bracelets had wiped all the info from the card. So, I had to take them off for the last five days. I was horrified and amazed that after two days of not wearing my stainless steel magnetic bracelets, the pain in my hands came back with a vengeance. As soon as I put them back on when I got home, I was further amazed at how quickly (only a couple of days) the pain eased and almost disappeared. This is truly a testimony to their worth–thank you"

Elizabeth Frith

"I purchased a magnetic back belt from you on 15th December and have worn it daily ever since, with amazing results. It has made a tremendous difference, not only to the level of pain I was experiencing, but to my general welfare as I am now far less stressed and have a much more positive outlook on the future—which at one time I was afraid to even consider what it might hold for me. I am highly delighted with the product and extol the virtue of magnet therapy to whoever will listen!"

J.Melling

"I am finding the magnetic water wand has reduced my blood pressure significantly—I am very pleased I bought it."

E. Wood, York

"I worked as a nurse many years ago. When I had my son 17 years ago I slipped a disc and was in absolute agony for years. I've suffered with spasms in my back ever since. I'm a very bubbly person, but when you're in constant pain you can't be bubbly and happy. I was fed up and depressed; the pain was there all the time. I was fed up with life—it got so bad.

After hearing Dee talk at a group meeting for the elderly, I volunteered to wear a back belt during the 2 hour session. At the end of the talk I could already feel a difference. I got a back belt and wore it constantly, only taking it off for a shower; you couldn't see it under my clothes. It has transformed my life. I am totally without pain. I swear by magnets. I've just found a way of controlling my pain. I very, very rarely take painkillers. I feel very lucky to have found a way out of my pain."

Denise Allen, aged 50, Derbyshire, Ex-nurse

Relieve Yourself Of Pain And Immobility In Just 7 Weeks Or Less

"I first heard about magnets years ago. My husband had terrible knees. He was very sceptical and didn't want to try it. I bought the knee straps and despite you saying that he wouldn't feel the benefits for a couple of weeks, he started to feel relief almost straight away and he continues to use them today.

I have carpal tunnel and have a bracelet for each wrist. I also have a back belt and knee straps and we sleep on a magnetic mattress cover. For my sciatica I have found all of these things very helpful and particularly with the carpal tunnel. I'm absolutely convinced that the magnets have helped me; they can't cure but they have helped with the pain."

Clare Gardener, aged 65, Nottinghamshire

"I suffered with arthritis for about 20 years. The last 5 years have been difficult. I've had trouble walking, moving about, and turning over in bed. Certain activity would spark off quite severe pain that I would basically have to live with for lengthy periods of time.

I was taking pain killers. I had physiotherapy and acupuncture which did help for a short time. My feet, toes, back and knees were pretty bad. I started with a back belt and a bed pad and started feeling the benefits after 2 to 3 weeks. The combination of all the things I have used has been the main contributing factor in my success. Sleeping on the mattress cover has helped me all over the body."

Christine Brooke, aged 61

"Over the 4-week period I've been using the magnets for my knee, I've stopped taking all my painkillers. I've gradually cut them down. People have told me that I am walking better and I feel that I am. I can definitely walk faster. When I went to see my doctor for a diabetes check up, he said 'you're not limping'. He wanted to know what I had done. He asked if I had increased my painkillers and I told him that I had actually stopped taking them. I took off my magnetic strap and showed it to him and he said to keep it on and carry on. He has now put my knee replacement on hold."

Jackie Mitchell

"My back problem goes back to 1948. I was playing football and someone shoulder-charged me. I slid on the ground and didn't think anything of it but when I came home and was sat down taking my muddy boots off, I just couldn't get back up again. The injury caused a curvature of the lower spine and any discs are now edge-shaped.

Now I keep my back belt on 24 hours a day and I sleep on the mattress cover. I have only been using it for 4 weeks and since then I don't get cramp in my legs during the night. I can get straight out of bed instead of easing myself out and hobbling along. I have niggles but nothing that bothers me. I am now spending 2 hours in the garden preparing the vegetable patch and I don't have any problems. I have been carrying around 75 litre bags of fertiliser without any twinges."

George Jennings

"I've tried acupuncture before and it didn't do anything for me. Now my back is a lot better. The only time my hip bothers me is when I've been shopping and sitting for a long time. I'm so pleased with the magnets. All of the fluid has gone out of my legs. My nurse is so pleased with the effects, and she thinks they are marvellous. I drink 4 glasses of magnetised water a day."

Iris Payne

"I'm not tossing and turning so much at night. I have the occasional restless night because of fibromyalgia, but in the main I am sleeping better. After just 2 days I noticed that I had energy, something that I don't normally have. It's hard to get out of bed but I wanted to wash my doors down.

Relieve Yourself Of Pain And Immobility In Just 7 Weeks Or Less

My husband normally does the housework because I can't manage it, but after 2 days of sleeping on the mattress cover I scrubbed down 3 doors, both sides, and I would never normally be able to do it. I'm feeling much brighter and my IBS is now under control. I'm very pleased."

Julia Leighton

"Since starting to use the magnets for my fibromyalgia, I'm sleeping a lot better and I feel a lot better. For the last 2 weeks my husband has been in hospital and I've been able to get to visit him everyday without pain or tiredness—my energy levels are better. The hospital is about 8 miles away and before the magnets I would never have even attempted to get there. I've had Fibromyalgia for 14 years and I think that I am coping a lot better now."

Yvonne Richardson

"I've had my magnetic package for one week and all of my pain has gone—I can't believe it. I've got arthritis in my spine from being run over years ago when I was little. I've had nagging, aching pain all my life. I was involved in a car crash 22 years ago and fractured my ribs and sternum. I'm wearing the magnets and drinking 6 glasses of the magnetised water a day and the pain has just gone, I can't believe it. My husband wants some now."

Valerie Sears

"After 4 weeks of use I still have some sciatica pain, but I think that's because I do a lot of lifting in my job. I wear the belt around my back all the time and I definitely feel that is has helped me and feel that it is going to carry on getting better."

Tina Smith

"After the first night of sleeping on the magnetic mattress cover, I woke up with more energy. The last 2 weeks I've had so much energy and have been catching up on my housework jobs. Most of my pain was in my back area and that's fine now. I'm sleeping better too. It's a pleasure now to go to bed, bedtime isn't my enemy now. I'm so happy with it— it's brilliant and I would recommend it to anyone!"

Sharon Heath, Fibromyalgia

"I have osteoporosis and I am waiting for an operation, but the waiting list is very long. Since starting to use my magnets I think my pain is about 50% less than it was before. I'm wearing the magnets all the time and drinking over 2 litres of magnetised water a day. I find that drinking it comes very naturally now; there is nothing to think about, you just drink it.

The pad, which I have in the bed, keeps my back so warm and comfortable throughout the night. It has made a huge difference and I will continue to use it. I am very happy with my progress!"

Diane Tunstall

"I really like the mattress cover. I'm sleeping a lot better. It certainly seems to help my Fibromyalgia. I've not been taking so many painkillers and when I do have pain, I lie on the mattress cover and it seems to ease it."

Lesley Dawson

"When I get out of bed the pain has been so much better, it's not totally gone but there's a big improvement. The mattress cover is so comfortable and in the morning I have so much more movement to push myself up and get out of bed. I'm not taking any painkillers now. I was taking Tramodol, but I don't take any now. I keep my small sleep pad in my chair downstairs and use it during the day. For me the biggest difference came when I started sleeping on the mattress cover"

Linda Milner, M.S.

Chapter six

There's A Difference Between 'Ordinary' Magnetic Therapy And <u>Clinical</u> Magnetic Therapy — Be Careful What You Use!

There are thousands of magnetic devices: straps, wraps, earrings, bracelets, necklaces and anklets that do nothing for you apart from take your money.

Here's the truth revealed:

'Ordinary' magnetic therapy professes two things. We now understand reasons for people not receiving pain relief with 'ordinary' magnetic therapy, and here they are:

Claim 1: That you just need to wear a magnetic bracelet around your wrist and it will take away the pain from any area of your body, no matter where your pain is, how severe it is or how long you have suffered with it.

Why it doesn't work: It's very simple: magnetic bracelets <u>cannot and will not</u> relieve pain in any of the flowing areas: knees, backs, feet, ankles, thighs, hips, shoulders and necks

<u>Or anywhere else on your body apart from your wrist, hand and fingers!</u>

I cannot emphasise the importance of understanding this point enough. In a nutshell, the action of magnets is only found locally around the area that they are placed.

There's A Difference Between 'Ordinary' Magnetic Therapy And Clinical Magnetic Therapy — Be Careful

The laws of physics prevent magnets working in any other way. It simply can't be because the very nature of a magnetic field is to act in this way.

Let me illustrate this point:

In 2006 a survey of 2596 people who purchased an 'ordinary' magnetic bracelet were asked what area of pain they were treating with the bracelet. The results were quite shocking:

- 883 were wearing the bracelet to treat back pain,
- 597 for wrist or hand pain,
- 545 for knee pain,
- 337 for neck pain,
- 260 for shoulder pain,
- 182 for foot pain.

The people wearing an 'ordinary' magnetic bracelet for pain in other areas other than the hand or wrist did not get any relief from their pain. And the vast majority, 2076 in fact, had either thrown their bracelet away or given it to someone else to try.

The most important lesson to take from this is to always wear magnets directly over your area of pain. By doing this you will give yourself the best chance of feeling a benefit.

Claim 2: You can place magnets around your area of pain if you wish but it doesn't matter what strength the magnets are, and you only need to wear them for a short period of time.

Why it doesn't work: Not all magnets are created equal. Making sure that you have the correct strength of magnet will be the difference between relieving pain and gaining absolutely no benefit whatsoever.

A minimum strength per magnet is required to ensure that the magnetic field is powerful enough to penetrate through the skin and into the bloodstream.

If a magnet does not have a minimum of 800 gauss (the unit of magnetic measurement is called gauss) then it will not penetrate into the skin.

The stronger the magnet, the deeper the penetration into the skin. So for more serious ailments and chronic, longstanding conditions, stronger magnets are recommended. 1,500-2,000 gauss magnets are considered to be high strength.

For extreme pain and very severe conditions super-strength magnets are advocated. These are magnets that have a gauss rating of 3,000 or above.

Super strength magnets are rapidly gaining in popularity as they such a deep level of penetration and create a very large magnetic field. Results are more rapid with this strength of magnet.

They are recommended for people who suffer with severe pain, for example from fibromyalgia, M.S., M.E. and severe arthritis.

A recent survey of people who have not benefited but are wearing magnets over their area of pain found that they are wearing weak magnets that were less than 800 gauss in strength, or they were wearing an 800 gauss magnet when the severity of their condition warrants a much stronger magnet.

Our advice for people is always the same: find out what strength of magnets you require, put the correct strength device directly over the area of pain and leave it in place 24 hours a day, 7 days a week until the pain has gone.

Claim 3: The bigger the magnet, the stronger it is. Or put another way, if your magnet can pick up a piece of cutlery it must be very strong.

There's A Difference Between 'Ordinary' Magnetic Therapy And Clinical Magnetic Therapy — Be Careful

Why it's not true: The size of a magnet is not relative to its strength; many magnetic suppliers claim that the bigger the magnet the stronger it will be; this is not the case. Very high-strength magnets, for example, a 3,000 gauss one can be as small as 3mm in diameter. Similarly, an 800 gauss magnet can be quite large, (in therapeutic terms) the size of a 2 pence piece. The smaller of the two magnets is by far the stronger. However a very simple 'sleight of hand' trick can be used (and I have seen it used more than once) to make you believe that the larger 800 gauss magnet is stronger than the smaller 3,000 gauss magnet. Here's how the 'trick' works:

The 800 gauss 2p sized magnet has a larger surface area than that of the 3mm 3,000 gauss magnet. This means that the 800 gauss magnet will cling to things, such as a fork or knife, more easily than the 3,000 gauss magnet. This has absolutely nothing to do with strength. It's simply a demonstration of surface area, and that does not equal penetration into the skin— remember: gauss is the unit of strength. The higher the number the stronger the magnet and the further it will penetrate into your tissues. This is what you should concern yourself with; not size.

The size of the magnet does determine one important factor, the range of the magnetic field. The larger the magnet the wider the spread of the magnetic field. This means that the field will radiate outwards in a wide circle, however it does not mean that the field will penetrate deep into the tissues. A small magnet will not create such a wide spread magnetic field surrounding the magnet but it will penetrate much deeper into the tissues.

The general rule to remember is:

1. A weak but large magnet will cover a large area on the skin, but will only have a shallow penetration depth into the skin.
2. A strong but small magnet will cover a small area on the skin, but will have a deep penetration depth into the skin.

To ensure that you have a wide magnetic field that also penetrates deep into the tissues, choose a magnet that is over 2,000 gauss and at least 8mm in diameter. The average size of a medical magnet is approximately 18mm in diameter.

Healing magnets are small because they have to be able to be placed as close to the point of injury as possible. If they were larger in size, it would not be easy to attach the magnets over the pain point. Plus, larger magnets are uncomfortable as they are heavy to wear and will "dig" into the skin.

Clinical Magnetic therapy works on the latest scientific principles which are:

Principle 1: Clinical magnets must be placed directly over the area of pain. If there are multiple-pain areas each area must be treated separately.

Why it works: A magnetic field only radiates a short distance. Think of it like the ripples on a pond: as you throw a stone into the water the ripples are very dense and tightly packed around the point of impact, but as the ripples spread out they get further apart and weaker until they disappear altogether.

The magnetic field works in the same manner in the body. The further away the magnet is from the area of pain, the weaker the strength of the magnetic field and the less benefit is felt.

The rule of thumb is very simple: place a magnetic device over each and every area of pain. If you have painful knees, back, hips and shoulders then you must wear a different device over each area. The magnet on your knee is not going to help your shoulder, back or hip. Each area of pain must be treated separately!

Principle 2: Clinical magnets must be an adequate strength for the type of condition, severity of the condition and the length of time the condition has been present.

There's A Difference Between 'Ordinary' Magnetic Therapy And Clinical Magnetic Therapy — Be Careful

Why it works: Every person's body reacts to substances, chemicals and electrical impulses in a slightly different way. Some people absorb a magnetic field very easily and rapidly, and will feel a very dramatic response in just a day or two. At the other end of the scale, a few people absorb a magnetic field very slowly, and they will find that they have to persevere for as long as 6 weeks before their body responds to the magnetic field.

The strength of magnet required for each individual is dependent on the type of ailment/injury, the severity and the length of time the ailment/injury has been there.

You cannot overdose by wearing too many magnets; there is no limit to the amount of magnetic strength that you can use at any one time.

The magnetic field created from a medical magnet can't harm the body. There is an electromagnetic current in all living things, including humans; it is essential for cellular function.

The magnetic field that flows from magnetic therapy devices is the same as the current that occurs naturally in our body.

As an example, an MRI (magnetic resonance imager) scanner used in hospitals for diagnosis purposes emits a magnetic field of around 450,000 gauss, (a medical magnet is usually a maximum of 3,000 gauss). People enter the scanner and have 450,000 gauss of magnetism forced through their body with absolutely no harmful effects.

Principle 3: Magnetised (ionised) water must be consumed in conjunction with placing clinical magnets over the area of pain. This is to ensure that the magnetic field that is circulating around the body has the same effect on the inside as the magnetic field has on the outside of the body.

Why it works: All water in its natural state (from rivers, streams, springs that has not been treated by chemicals) is naturally magnetised. This is because the Earth itself is a gigantic magnet (gravity is a magnetic field) with a north and a south pole. All water, before it is treated, is magnetically charged by the Earth's magnetic field.

The water that comes out of the tap has been chemically treated and transported in lead pipes; this destroys the naturally-occurring magnetisation (also called ionisation) in the water.

By introducing a water magnet (shaped like a stick with a ball on the end) to your tap, filtered or bottled water for 15 minutes, you re-magnetise the water and with it gain its substantial benefits.

Just 4 glasses a day is enough to see quite dramatic differences in a person's pain levels, but it can't be used alone. It must be used in conjunction with magnets directly over the area of pain.

It can't harm you and does not interfere with any medications or treatments. It does not alter your body in anyway.

Magnetised water has several beneficial properties:
- It aids absorption of nutrients from our food,
- It aids digestion,
- It detoxifies the blood,
- It regulates hormone levels; particularly insulin, serotonin, melatonin and endorphin,
- It lowers high blood pressure
- It increases the strength of the magnetic field at the point of pain
- It also speeds up the healing process by increasing the absorption rate of the magnetic field by up to an amazing 6-10 times.

Principle 4: Clinical magnetic therapy should be used 24 hours a day and 7 days a week until the pain has completely subsided and full mobility is regained.

There's A Difference Between 'Ordinary' Magnetic Therapy And Clinical Magnetic Therapy — Be Careful

Why it works: The magnets begin to work the moment you first place them on, and as you keep them in place day and night it will only be a matter of 3-6 weeks on average before pain relief is felt.

What will happen is that the magnetic field starts to reduce inflammation (swelling) and increase endorphin levels (the body's own painkillers), to regain mobility and movement.

Over a period of days, or a few weeks, the benefits gradually increase. As long as the magnets are left in place day and night, this process happens in 93% of people who are using the correct device and strength for their pain.

It's natural be impatient, and we all seem to live in a world of instant gratification, where we want results instantly.

With clinical magnetic therapy, however, you must be prepared to have a little patience and wait a short while for the results to become evident.

If you take the magnets off after just a day or two, then no benefit or relief whatsoever will be felt.

Principle 5: Most importantly clinical magnets must be used throughout the night.

Why it works: When you think about it logically, sleeping on magnets makes a lot of sense. When we are asleep our body automatically slows down our heart rate and respiration rate; we enter into a rest phase so our body doesn't need so much energy to function.

The excess resources of oxygen and nutrients, that are available during sleep, are sent straight to the areas that need them the most, namely injured areas. It is at night-time when most of your body's healing takes place.

Sleeping on magnets actually stimulates and enhances this natural process. The magnets dramatically boost the body's natural healing process, reducing the time it takes for your pain to be resolved and for your mobility to be increased.

They regulate the sleep hormone melatonin, promoting deep and restful sleep. They leave the user rested and energised on waking in the morning.

A recent survey which compared the success-rate of 'ordinary' magnetic therapy with clinical magnetic therapy revealed that only 30% of 'ordinary' magnetic therapy users reported any pain loss or improved mobility. Whereas those using clinical magnetic therapy showed a 93% success rate of pain-reduction and regained mobility.

You must understand that if you have tried 'ordinary' magnetic therapy and it didn't work for you, you shouldn't dismiss clinical magnetic therapy altogether because there is a very strong possibility that you were not using the correct magnet for your needs, and the correct application of clinical magnetic therapy will work.

Chapter Seven

Now It's Your Turn: Relieve Your Pain, Regain Your Mobility And Get Your Life Back Again

My one and only mission is to help you understand that there is something that can help you; <u>that pain relief is real.</u>

You can be rid of your pain without taking pills, injections or visits to physiotherapists, chiropractics, pain clinics etc. Have the rest of your life without pain and with your full mobility reinstated. Enjoy life more than you ever have since developing your condition.

I know it's real because I have personally come through extreme pain and suffering, as a result of severe injuries, to the point of having no pain and complete mobility today.

Life is, once more, wonderful and free. This is why today I now have a passion to share this method of relieving pain and immobility and achieving what seemed to be a 'miraculous' turnaround with you.

I know this through 7 years of my own experience, plus through the experience of thousands of people who have contacted us after undergoing clinical magnetic therapy who are now free of pain and have regained mobility. Clinical magnetic therapy is a wonderful and effective relief for arthritis, back pain, fibromyalgia, osteoporosis, multiple sclerosis, stroke, Spondylosis and joint pain.

It's my mission in life to help as many people like you be rid of pain and to have mobility restored.

Relieve Yourself Of Pain And Immobility In Just 7 Weeks Or Less

This breakthrough in clinical magnetic therapy enables you to feel your pain disappear and your mobility returning. You will be so delighted; life will be colourful and free again.

I have arranged for every reader of this book to have a trial person-alised clinical magnetic therapy treatment pack with absolutely no risk for an unusually long 180 days. Within those 180 days, your pain and swelling is virtually guaranteed to be relieved.

See the personal 180 day risk-free trial letter enclosed.

I can assure you as a pain nurse with more than 14 years of experience within the NHS there is an answer to your pain problem, and the answer can relieve you of even the most severe pain within just days or a few short weeks.

Don't leave your pain one more day without applying the virtually magic effects of clinical magnetic therapy.

Finally...

My greatest wish is that you will now not do yourself the disservice of being satisfied with the pain and immobility you are suffering from at this very moment.

My wish is that you will now actually embrace the powerful message that I have shared with you in this book through my own experience and the experiences of the 69 people who shared their stories with you

And that you will truly take positive action in taking control of your pain and immobility by just giving it a try. Surely its worth a little bit of time and patience just to try it; of course it is. You can get your life back, and if I'm wrong you don't lose anything. You're protected and safe with us. We are nurses, we really do care and are always here to help in every way we can.

Now It's Your Turn: Relieve Your Pain, Regain Your Mobility And Get Your Life Back Again

If you wake up tomorrow morning and you haven't ordered your personalised clinical magnetic therapy pack, you will have to live with the fact that the pain you are suffering with will carry on.

But if you wake up tomorrow morning realising that you have done something about it, you will be joyous in the knowledge that in a very short period of time your pain is virtually guaranteed to be relieved. You can live a lifetime from now free of pain with your mobility restored. Do it now; don't leave it a moment longer.

My very best wishes to you, and I hope to see you through your pain to a pain-free and more mobile way of life.